About the NCCN Guidelines for Patients®

National Comprehensive Cancer Network®

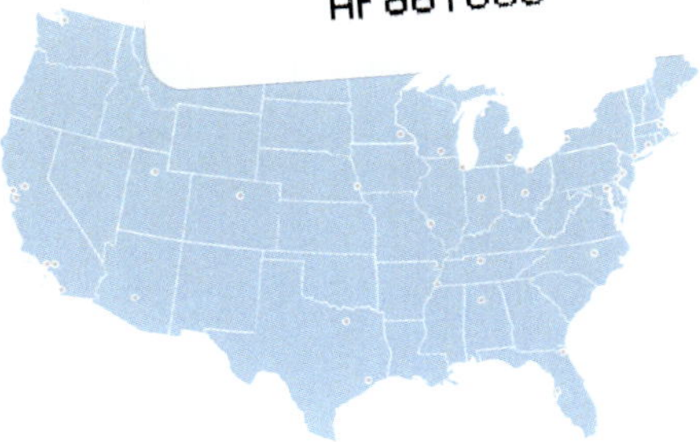

Did you know that top cancer centers across the United States work together to improve cancer care? This alliance of leading cancer centers is called the National Comprehensive Cancer Network® (NCCN®).

Cancer care is always changing. NCCN develops evidence-based cancer care recommendations used by health care providers worldwide. These frequently updated recommendations are the NCCN Clinical Practice Guidelines in Oncology (NCCN Guidelines®). The NCCN Guidelines for Patients plainly explain these expert recommendations for people with cancer and caregivers.

These NCCN Guidelines for Patients are based on the NCCN Clinical Practice Guidelines in Oncology (NCCN Guidelines®) for NCCN Clinical Guidelines for Basal Cell Skin Cancer, Version 1.2025 – January 17, 2025.

View the NCCN Guidelines for Patients free online
NCCN.org/patientguidelines

Find an NCCN Cancer Center near you
NCCN.org/cancercenters

Connect with us

Supporters

NCCN Guidelines for Patients are supported by funding from the NCCN Foundation®

NCCN Foundation gratefully acknowledges the following corporate supporter for helping to make available these NCCN Guidelines for Patients: Regeneron Pharmaceuticals, Inc.

NCCN independently adapts, updates, and hosts the NCCN Guidelines for Patients. Our corporate supporters do not participate in the development of the NCCN Guidelines for Patients and are not responsible for the content and recommendations contained therein.

To make a gift or learn more, visit online or email

NCCNFoundation.org/donate

PatientGuidelines@NCCN.org

Contents

NCCN Foundation seeks to support the millions of patients and their families affected by a cancer diagnosis by funding and distributing NCCN Guidelines for Patients. NCCN Foundation is also committed to advancing cancer treatment by funding the nation's promising doctors at the center of innovation in cancer research. For more details and the full library of patient and caregiver resources, visit NCCN.org/patients.

National Comprehensive Cancer Network (NCCN) and NCCN Foundation
3025 Chemical Road, Suite 100, Plymouth Meeting, PA 19462 USA

1

About basal cell skin cancer

Basal cell skin cancer, also known as basal cell carcinoma (BCC), is the most common type of skin cancer. About 3 million cases of basal cell skin cancer are diagnosed every year in the United States. The good news is it can be cured in most cases. Treatment usually involves surgery to remove the cancer. Keep reading to find out more.

What is basal cell skin cancer?

Basal cell skin cancer is the most common of all skin cancer types. If caught early, it is easily treatable and curable. This is because it rarely metastasizes (spreads).

Skin cancers often occur in the top layer of the skin (epidermis) and less commonly in the middle layer of the skin (dermis). The epidermis is made up of basal cells and other cells. Basal cell skin cancer occurs when some basal cells become abnormal and grow out of control. This cancer usually develops in areas exposed to the sun, including the face, head, neck, arms, legs, and trunk. But it can occur anywhere on the body.

Skin lesions

Basal cell skin cancer is often found on the face, head, and neck. Here is a basal cell lesion pictured on a person's cheek.

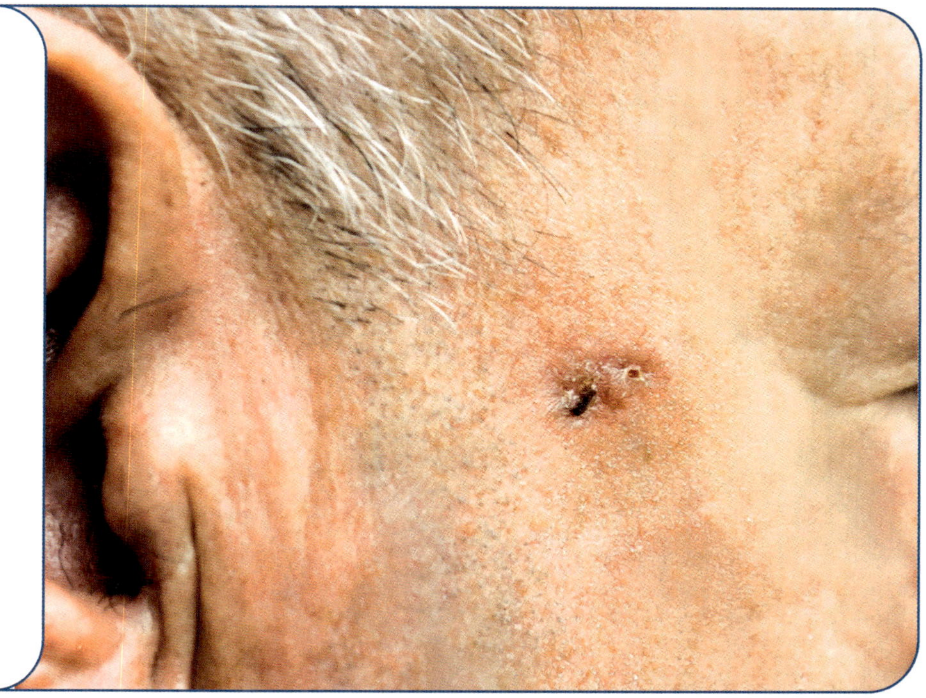

Skin basics

Did you know that your skin is your body's largest organ and if you measured it it would stretch to about 20 square feet?

Working as a barrier, your skin protects you from bacteria and chemicals and helps control your body temperature. It has 3 layers:

- **Epidermis** – The top layer of skin provides a waterproof barrier and creates skin color (melanin).
- **Dermis** – The middle layer involves connective tissue, blood vessels, oil and sweat glands, nerves, and hair follicles.
- **Hypodermis** – The deepest tissue layer is made up of fat and connective tissue.

Most skin cancers form in the cells of the epidermis. It has 3 main types of cells:

- **Squamous cells** – These cells are flat cells found in the upper part of the epidermis.
- **Basal cells** – Found in the lower part of the epidermis, basal cells constantly divide to form new cells that replace the squamous cells on the skin's surface.
- **Melanocytes** – Melanocytes are cells located in the lower part of the epidermis that produce melanin. Melanin is responsible for our hair, skin, and eye color. It also protects our skin from harmful ultraviolet (UV) rays.

Skin layers and cell types

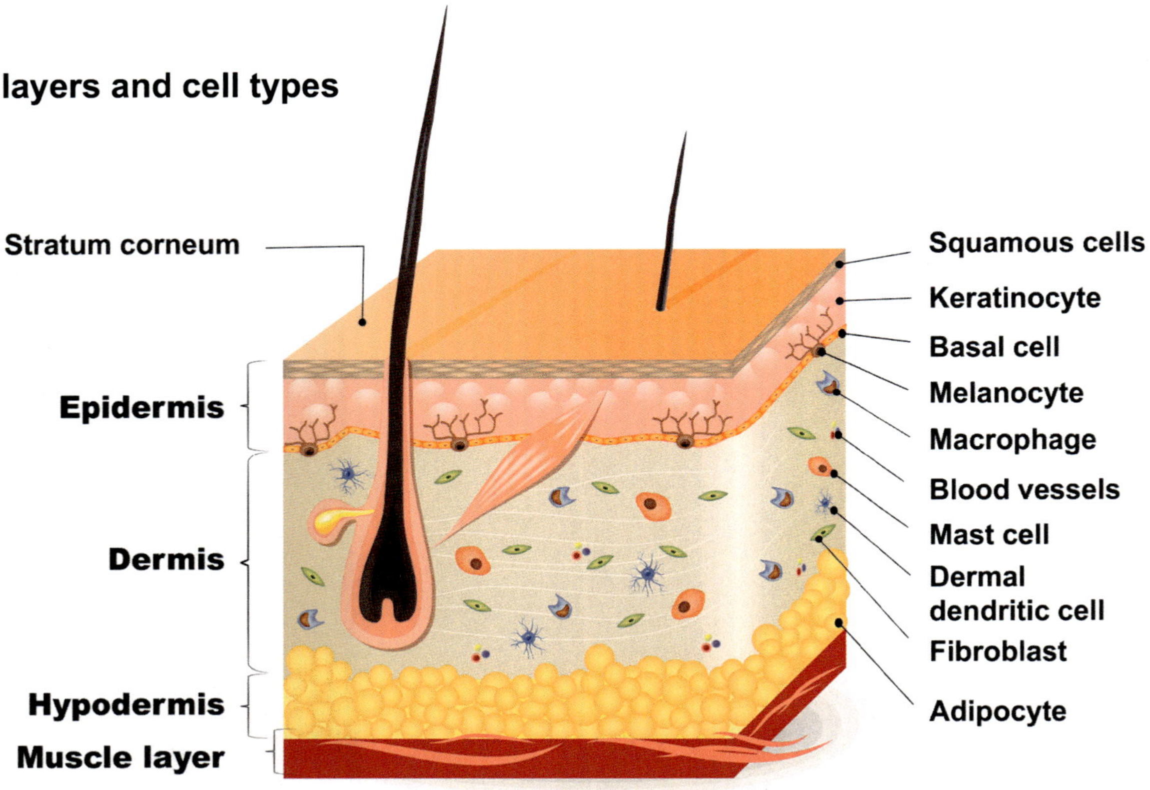

This book is only about basal cell skin cancer. For more information on squamous cell skin cancer or melanoma, read the *NCCN Guidelines for Patients*, available at NCCN.org/patientguidelines and on the NCCN Patient Guides for Cancer app.

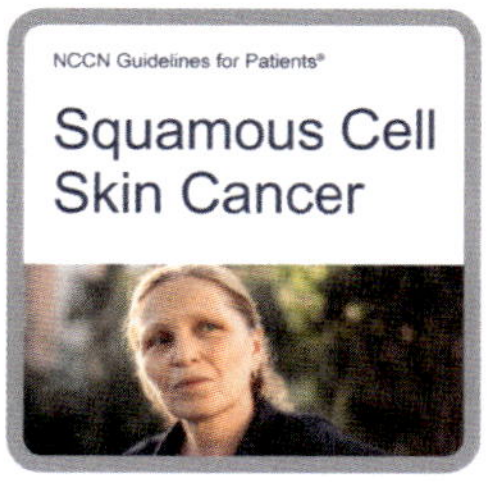

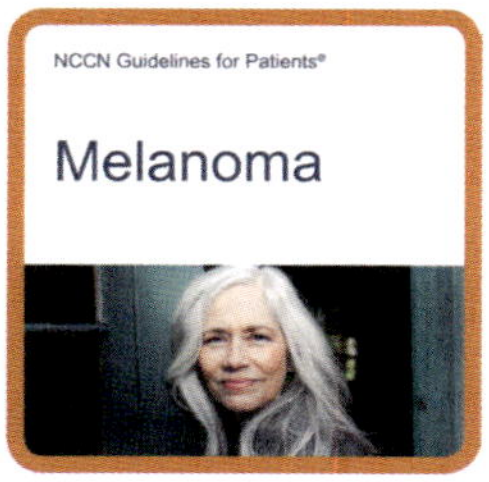

Signs and symptoms

Basal cell skin cancer can happen to anyone but it's most common in people with lighter skin, lighter hair, or lighter eyes. In lighter skin, its lesions can look like any of the following:

- Flat, pale or yellow areas, like a scar
- Red patches that might be itchy
- Small, pink or red, shiny bumps that may have blue, brown, or black areas
- Open sores that don't heal and might bleed, or go away and come back

In darker (brown and black) skin, basal cell skin cancer can appear as a brown or glossy black bump with a rolled border. It can be mistaken for a normal mole.

Be sure to look out for any new, changing, bleeding, or unusual skin growths. Skin cancer is easier to cure when it is caught early.

To find out how basal cell skin cancer is diagnosed, read *Chapter 2: Testing for basal cell skin cancer.*

Causes and risk factors

Basal cell skin cancer is caused by exposure to UV radiation from the sun or other sources like tanning beds. UV radiation can harm the DNA inside basal skin cells. DNA controls how cells grow and function. If the DNA inside cells becomes damaged, the cells can become abnormal and grow out of control.

You're more likely to have basal cell skin cancer if you have certain risk factors. A risk factor increases the chance of developing cancer. Risk factors for basal cell skin cancer include:

- **UV light exposure** – UV light (radiation) that comes from the sun or tanning beds increases your risk.
- **Fair skin, red or blond hair, or light eye color** – People with lighter-colored skin are at a higher risk of developing skin cancer because melanin (skin pigment) filters out the sun's harmful UV rays.
- **Age** – Risk increases with age because sun exposure builds up over time. But skin cancer is becoming more common in younger people.
- **History of skin cancer** – If you or someone in your family has had skin cancer, you're more likely to develop any type of skin cancer.
- **Radiation therapy** – Radiation treatment for other conditions, especially at a young age, can cause skin cancer.
- **Immune suppression** – People with weakened immune systems from organ transplants or autoimmune diseases are at higher risk for basal cell skin cancer.

How is basal cell skin cancer treated?

Basal cell skin cancer is highly treatable and curable. Catching it and treating it early is key.

Surgery is the most common treatment for basal cell skin cancer. In some cases, radiation therapy or systemic therapy might be used to treat it.

Following your treatment, you will have full skin exams with your doctor at least once a year. Between these periods, prevention is important. See *Chapter 4: Treatment by risk and recurrence* for more information.

Recurrence is when basal cell skin cancer returns to the area where it was originally found, or it has metastasized (spread) to the lymph nodes or to distant parts of the body. But there are several options for how to treat it.

Read more about how your cancer is treated in *Chapter 3: Types of treatment* and *Chapter 4: Treatment by risk and recurrence*.

What can you do to get the best care?

Advocate for yourself. You have an important role to play in your care. In fact, you're more likely to get the care you want by asking questions and making shared decisions with your care team.

The NCCN Guidelines for Patients will help you understand cancer care. With better understanding, you'll be more prepared to discuss your care with your team and share your concerns. Many people feel more satisfied when they play an active role in their care.

You may not know what to ask your care team. That's common. Each chapter in this book ends with an important section called *Questions to ask.* These suggested questions will help you get more information on all aspects of your care.

Take the next step and keep reading to learn what is the best care for you!

Why you should read this resource

Making decisions about cancer care can be stressful. You may need to make tough decisions under pressure about complex choices.

The NCCN Guidelines for Patients are trusted by patients and providers. They clearly explain current care recommendations made by respected experts in the field. Recommendations are based on the latest research and practices at leading cancer centers.

Cancer care is not the same for everyone. By following expert recommendations for your situation, you are more likely to improve your care and have better outcomes as a result. Use this book as your guide to find the information you need to make important decisions.

2

Testing for basal cell skin cancer

Treatment planning starts with testing. Accurate testing is needed to diagnose and then treat basal cell skin cancer. This chapter presents an overview of the tests you might receive and what to expect.

Whether you or your doctor found a concerning lesion on your skin, testing is needed to identify and diagnose basal cell skin cancer. The diagnosis is based on the results in your medical and family history, a physical exam, skin exam, and biopsy, and, in some cases, imaging studies. **See Guide 1**. Your diagnosis will determine your treatment plan. It is important you understand what these tests mean, so keep reading for more details.

Guide 1
Common tests for basal cell skin cancer

Medical and family history
Physical exam
Complete skin exam
Biopsy
Imaging tests (for lesions that might have spread)

General health tests

Medical history

A medical history is a record of all health issues and treatments you have had in your life. Be prepared to list any illness or injury and when it happened. Bring a list of old and new medicines and any over-the-counter medicines, herbals, or supplements you take. Tell your health care provider about any symptoms you have. A medical history will help determine which treatment is best for you.

Family history

Some cancers and other diseases can run in families. Your provider will ask about the health history of family members who are blood relatives. This information is called a family history. Ask your family members about their health issues like heart disease, cancer, and diabetes, and at what age they were diagnosed.

Physical exam

During a physical exam, a health care provider may:

- Look in your eyes, ears, nose, and throat
- Feel and apply pressure to parts of your body to see if organs are of normal size, are soft or hard, or cause pain when touched
- Feel for enlarged lymph nodes in your neck, underarm, and groin
- Conduct a complete skin exam

Skin exam

It is important to find an experienced health care provider, like a dermatologist, to perform a thorough skin exam. The skin is your body's largest organ. Not only does it protect your body, but it tells doctors a lot about your health.

Expect a head-to-toe skin exam that includes review of the scalp, face, mouth, eyes and eyelids, ears, neck, trunk, arms, hands, fingers, fingernails, feet, toes, and toenails.

Your provider may use a dermatoscope (see photo) to see spots more clearly.

Lesion

A skin lesion is defined as an area of skin that looks different than the surrounding area. When it comes to skin cancer, it's also referred to as a tumor. This can include an abnormal spot, lump, bump, ulcer, sore, or colored area of the skin. Most lesions are harmless, but some may be skin cancer. Speak to your provider or care team about any lesions that have changed in color, texture, or growth.

Skin color

You know your skin better than anyone. Tell your provider about your normal skin color. Show where the skin looks normal and where it looks different to you. Describe any changes. The risk for skin cancer is higher among those with lighter skin color but anyone can develop basal cell skin cancer.

Skin exam

A doctor may use a dermatoscope (a special magnifying lens and light source held near the skin) to get a closer look at spots.

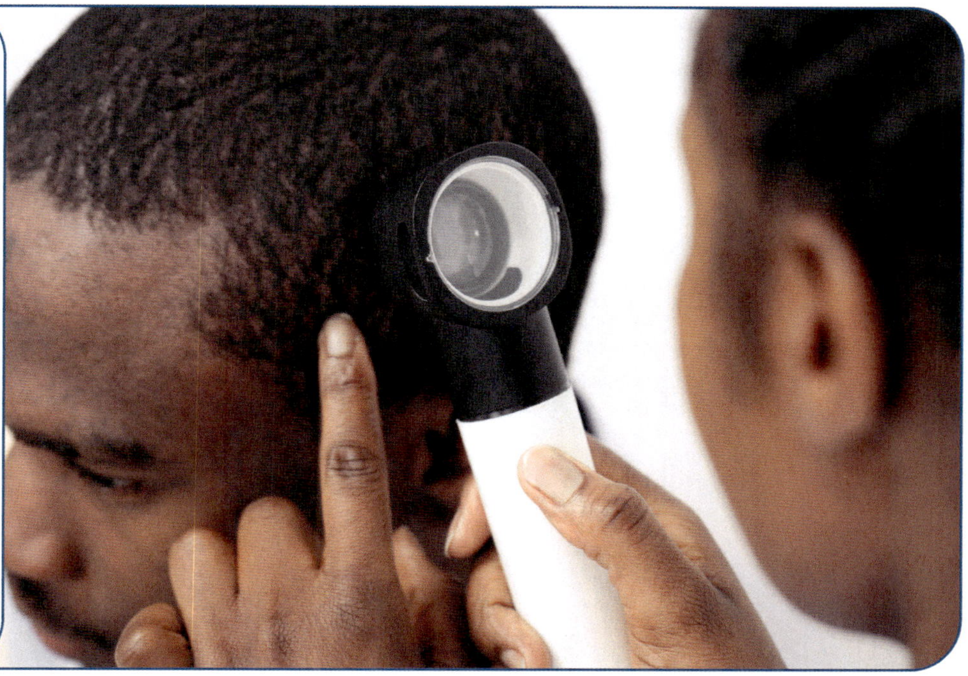

Biopsy

A skin biopsy starts when an unusual lesion is found on your skin. Your provider will remove some or all of it and send it to a lab to be tested for cancer.

It's important to note that biopsy is not the same as having surgery. The point of biopsy is diagnosis. The point of surgery is to remove the lesion and have its margins examined. For more information on surgery, read *Chapter 3: Types of treatment*.

What happens during biopsies

Your provider will numb the area first with a local anesthetic. This will likely be through an injection with a small needle. While you might feel some minor pain from the anesthetic, it prevents you from feeling any pain with the biopsy.

Because cutting the skin is involved with the biopsy, a scar is likely to occur. You may want to ask how the biopsy incision will be closed. There are a few options including stitches or a special glue that can be used. Be sure to talk to your provider about your concerns with scarring.

For basal cell skin cancer, three types of biopsies are commonly used: excisional, skin punch, or shave.

Excisional biopsy

During an excisional biopsy, all or part of the lesion may be removed. This biopsy can be done in a doctor's office or at a hospital. If the lesion is small and shallow enough, it may be removed entirely during the biopsy. Stitches are often used to close the wound.

Skin punch biopsy

In a skin punch biopsy, a small piece of skin and connective tissue are removed using a

Skin punch biopsy

Pictured are 2 punch biopsies to test for skin cancer before being closed.

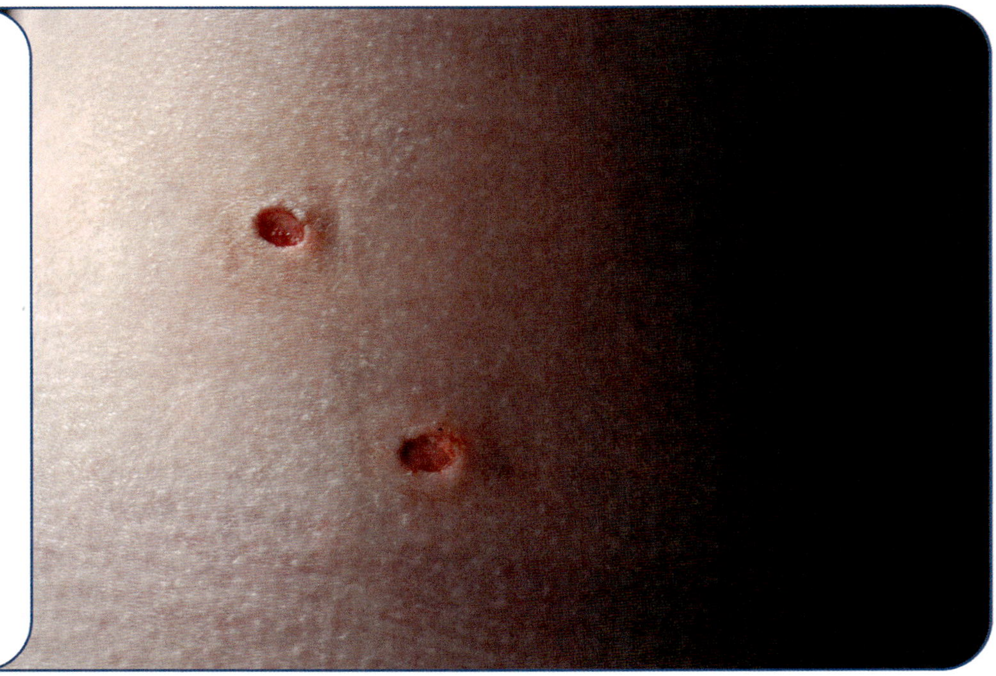

hand-held tool. Stitches are often used to close the opening in the skin made by the biopsy.

Shave biopsy

With a shave biopsy, a sharp blade or scalpel is used to "shave off" a thin layer of skin from the lesion. To help with bleeding, the doctor may apply an ointment, a chemical, or small electrical current to cauterize the area.

Biopsy testing

Your sample will be sent to a lab and will be reviewed by a pathologist. The pathologist will note the overall appearance and the size, shape, and type of your cells.

Imaging

Imaging tests take pictures (images) of the inside of your body. An imaging test is not typically needed for basal cell skin cancer unless it is very large and deep. These tests are usually used to see what tissues the cancer might have spread into, either deeper or farther away in the body.

CT scan

A computed tomography (CT or CAT) scan is a computerized x-ray machine. It takes many pictures (x-rays) from different angles of the same body part. Pictures are merged to form a 3D image.

MRI scan

A magnetic resonance imaging (MRI) scan uses strong magnets and radio waves to take digital pictures of the inside of the body. It does not use x-rays.

What's next

This chapter gave an overview of the different types of tests, from skin exams to imaging, that are used to diagnose basal cell skin cancer. Now that you know the kinds of tests you might have, read the next chapter on the variety of treatments available. To find out more specifically how your cancer might be treated, read *Chapter 4: Treatment by risk and recurrence*.

> **"I've had people tell me that it's just skin cancer like it's no big deal. People don't know how serious skin cancers like basal cell skin cancer can be."**

Key points

- Different types of testing like a physical exam, skin exam, and skin biopsy are needed to diagnose basal cell skin cancer.
- During your skin exam, your provider will examine your skin for unusual lesions and will keep track of any spots that need to be watched or checked more closely.
- If an unusual lesion is found on your skin, part of it or all of it will be removed and sent to a lab and tested for cancer. This is called a skin biopsy.
- Imaging is used to get a clearer picture of any evidence of spread. It is not commonly used for most basal cell skin cancer except when the cancer is advanced.

Questions to ask

- Why did I get this specific test?
- Do I need other tests to confirm my diagnosis?
- How deep and wide will the biopsy go into my skin?
- Will the wound be closed with stiches?
- How much scarring will there be from the biopsy?

3

Types of treatment

This chapter presents an overview of the types of treatment for basal cell skin cancer and what to expect. Most often some form of surgery is used to remove the cancerous lesion. Keep in mind not everyone will receive the same treatment.

Treatment options for basal cell skin cancer aim to remove the cancer completely. These include surgery, topical treatments, radiation therapy, and sometimes systemic (whole-body) treatment. Treatment received through a clinical trial may also be an option. But the most common treatment is surgery to remove the cancer and some of the healthy tissue around it. **See Guide 2**.

Guide 2 Common treatments for basal cell skin cancer
Surgery
Topical treatments
Radiation therapy
Systemic therapy
Clinical trials

Surgery

Surgical treatments include surgical excision, Mohs surgery, curettage and electrodesiccation, and shave removal:

Surgical excision

A surgical excision means cutting out the skin cancer along with some normal-looking tissue around it (surgical margin) to make sure all the cancer cells are removed. A local anesthetic will be used to numb the area before the surgery. A local anesthetic is the medicine that numbs a small area of the body to minimize pain. The lesion will be sent to the lab, also referred to as pathology. There, it will be analyzed for cancer.

After surgery, your doctor may close the opening (incision) with stitches. If the opening is large, you may require a skin graft. A skin graft takes skin from an unaffected area of the body to cover damaged skin. Common side effects of skin grafts include pain, swelling, bleeding, scarring, and infection.

PDEMA

A peripheral and deep en face margin assessment (PDEMA) refers to a technique that allows your doctor to view a high-quality image of the entire marginal surface of removed tissues. This may also be called a complete margin assessment. The most common form of PDEMA is Mohs micrographic surgery.

Mohs micrographic surgery

Mohs micrographic surgery, often referred to as Mohs surgery, is commonly used to remove a lesion (sometimes called a tumor) and the least amount of normal tissue from the skin.

Mohs surgery involves many stages:

- First, your doctor will mark the area to be removed (including the tumor).
- Your doctor will then numb the area with a local anesthetic and use a scalpel to remove a thin layer of the tumor.
- Next, the tissue sample will be evaluated at an on-site lab. At this time, your tumor will be analyzed while you wait.

If there are additional areas of concern around the edges or base of the tissue sample, you will go back to the operating space for another round of tissue removal. You will continue this process until all of the affected area has been removed.

Once no remaining cancer is found, your doctor will decide the best option to close the opening. In some cases, the surgical opening can heal on its own. But most of the time, stitches are used.

Mohs surgery is generally considered safe and carries a low risk of complications. But there are some potential side effects that include bleeding and bruising, infection, pain, numbness, swelling, and scarring.

Mohs surgery

Mohs surgery is very effective for treating basal cell skin cancer. The surgeon removes thin layers of skin — one at a time — and checks each layer for cancer until all the cancer cells are gone.

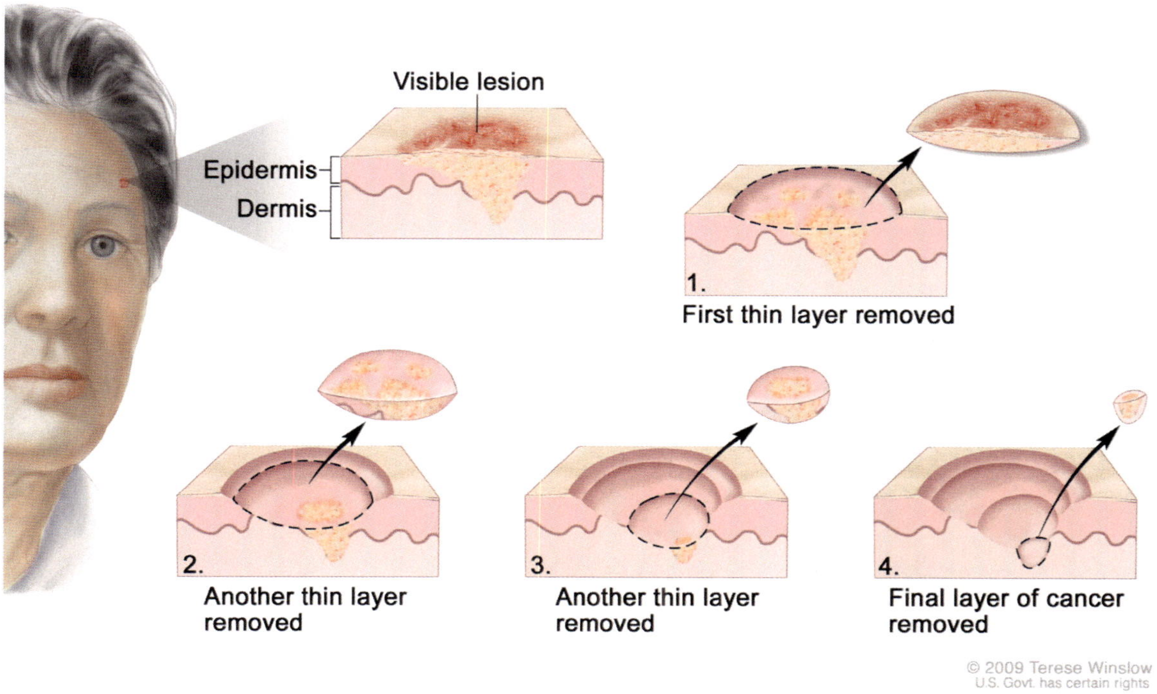

Curettage and electrodesiccation

Curettage and electrodesiccation is a procedure used to remove shallow (superficial) skin cancers and pre-cancers. During this procedure, your doctor will inject a local anesthetic into the affected area to numb it. Then the lesion will be removed by scraping it with a special tool that has a sharp looped edge on one side (a curette). Once the affected area is removed, it will be cauterized (burned) with electrical currents (known as electrodesiccation) to control the bleeding and destroy any remaining lesion.

The curettage and electrodesiccation procedure may be repeated if the growth is cancerous. This treatment can be an option for people who cannot undergo more invasive surgeries.

Curettage and electrodesiccation can cause side effects like pain, swelling, crusting or bleeding, and scarring.

Shave removal

This technique treats skin lesions that are raised or in the upper layer of the skin. Your doctor will numb the area and use a small blade to remove the outer layers of skin. The removed area includes all or part of the lesion.

Stitches are usually not needed. After the procedure, medicine is applied to stop any bleeding, or the area may be cauterized to seal blood vessels.

Potential side effects of shave removal include pain, bleeding, swelling, and infection.

Basal cell scar after treatment

Pictured here is a person's skin after basal cell skin cancer has been removed with surgery. Speak to your doctor about how your skin will be closed after your procedure and what the scar may look like.

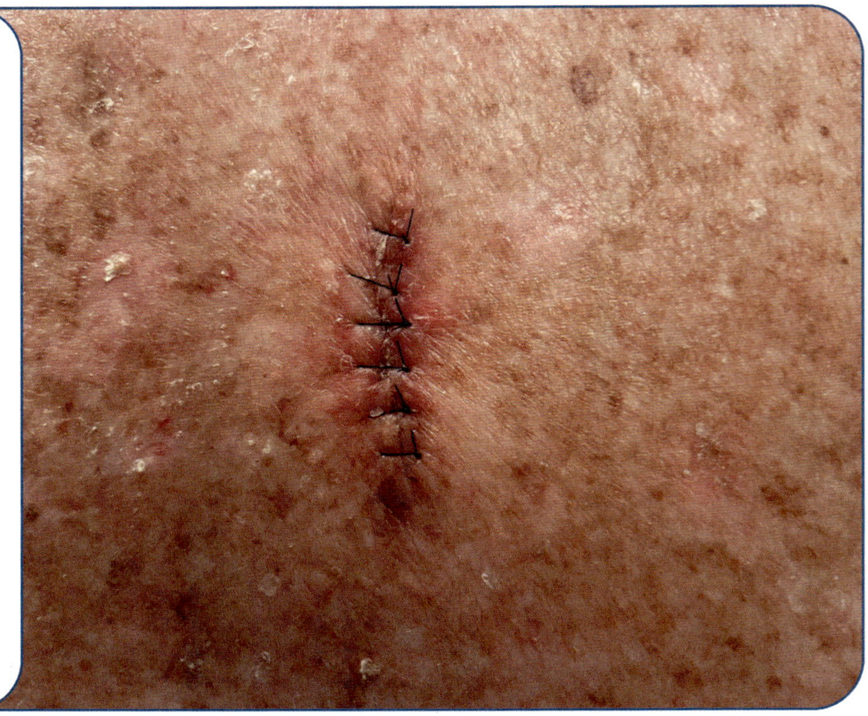

Topical treatments

Chemotherapy

Chemotherapy kills fast-growing cells throughout the body, including cancer cells and normal cells. All chemotherapies stop cancer cells from growing and dividing. You might think chemotherapy is given only through infusion, injection, or by mouth. But it can also come in a topical form applied on the skin. For treatment of basal cell skin cancer, the following topical chemotherapy creams may be used:

- Imiquimod (Aldara)
- Fluorouracil (Carac, Efudex, Fluoroplex)

Common side effects include red, blistering, itchy, or painful skin where the topical treatment is applied and can last a few days to weeks after treatment.

Cryotherapy

Cryotherapy (also called cryosurgery) freezes and destroys precancerous and cancerous tissue using a very cold liquid that is sprayed on the area. Liquid nitrogen is often used. Cryotherapy sometimes causes a burning sensation during treatment. A blister and scab will form, which heals over 2 to 3 weeks. Skin darkening or lightening can happen while it is healing.

Photodynamic therapy

In photodynamic therapy (PDT), a light-sensitive drug is applied to the area. When exposed to light (either red or blue light in the doctor's office, or shaded outdoor light), the drug becomes active and kills cancer cells. Common side effects of PDT include itching or burning when the liquid is applied, pain during the red or blue light exposure, and itching and redness for a few days after treatment.

Your care team

With basal cell skin cancer, you may only need to see your dermatologist for treatment. But depending on your diagnosis, your treatment team could include the following specialists:

Mohs surgeons are board-certified dermatologists with extra training in Mohs surgery and skin reconstruction. They specialize in surgical treatment and repair of skin cancers.

Surgical oncologists are doctors who are trained to diagnose and surgically treat and remove cancerous tumors.

Medical oncologists are doctors who specialize in prescribing cancer drugs. They are trained to diagnose and treat cancer using special medicines that may be taken by mouth or given through a vein.

Radiation oncologists are doctors who are trained to use different types of radiation to destroy cancerous cells while keeping other cells healthy.

Pathologists are doctors who are trained to study tissue and cells removed during a biopsy under a microscope to determine the risk status of a lesion.

Plastic surgeons are doctors who reconstruct, restore, and repair body parts. They may be needed to close a wound after surgery, especially if it involves deeper tissue.

Radiation therapy

Radiation therapy uses radiation from electrons, photons, protons, or other sources to kill cancer cells and shrink tumors. To treat skin cancers, low-energy photons or electron beam radiation are often used through a machine outside the body to send radiation toward the lesion. These types of radiation only penetrate the skin, making them effective at targeting cancer cells while minimizing damage to deeper tissues. Treatment may focus on individual lesions, a small area of the body, or specific lymph nodes. Radiation therapy can be given alone or with other treatments. For example, it can be used before, during, or after surgery to treat or slow the growth of cancer, especially if the surgical margin has cancer cells.

One other type of radiation that is less commonly used is brachytherapy. This is a type of radiation that can be helpful to treat basal cell skin cancers on the head and neck. It uses an applicator that's placed on top of the tumor or inside of it to deliver the radiation.

Common side effects of radiation therapy can include temporary fatigue, skin irritation (redness, blistering, and peeling) typically limited to the treated area, and changes in skin color.

What are targeted therapy and immunotherapy?

Targeted therapy is a cancer treatment that uses medicine to focus on specific molecules involved in cancer growth. By interfering with these molecules, it helps to slow or stop the spread of cancer cells.

Immunotherapy helps your immune system fight cancer. There are several types, but some of the most common are immune checkpoint inhibitors and monoclonal antibodies. Each type works to enhance your body's natural defenses against cancer.

Systemic therapy

Systemic therapy is a cancer treatment that affects the whole body. It is mainly used for advanced basal cell skin cancer.

Systemic therapies include targeted therapy, immunotherapy, and, in rare cases, systemic chemotherapy. Each therapy works differently to shrink the tumor and prevent recurrence.

Systemic therapies used to treat advanced basal cell skin cancer include:

- **Vismodegib (Erivedge)** – Vismodegib is a targeted therapy that is given orally. Common side effects can include muscle spasm, fatigue, hair loss, altered taste, and weight loss.
- **Sonidegib (Odomzo)** – Sonidegib is a targeted therapy that is given orally. Common side effects include diarrhea, abdominal pain, weight loss, hair loss, fatigue, and altered taste.
- **Cemiplimab-rwlc (Libtayo)** – Cemiplimab-rwlc is an immunotherapy. It is given as a 30-minute intravenous

(IV) infusion usually in a hospital or clinic. Common side effects include constipation, hair loss, and muscle, bone, back, and joint pain.

Clinical trials

A clinical trial is a type of medical research study. After being developed and tested in a lab, potential new ways of fighting cancer need to be studied in people.

If found to be safe and effective in a clinical trial, a drug, device, or treatment approach may be approved by the U.S. Food and Drug Administration (FDA). Everyone with cancer should carefully consider all of the treatment options available for their cancer type, including standard treatments and clinical trials. Talk to your doctor about whether a clinical trial may make sense for you.

Phases

Most cancer clinical trials focus on treatment and are done in phases.

- **Phase 1** trials study the safety and side effects of an investigational drug or treatment approach.
- **Phase 2** trials study how well the drug or approach works against a specific type of cancer.
- **Phase 3** trials test the drug or approach against a standard treatment. If the results are good, it may be approved by the FDA.
- **Phase 4** trials study the safety and benefit of an FDA-approved treatment.

Finding a clinical trial

In the United States

NCCN Cancer Centers
NCCN.org/cancercenters

The National Cancer Institute (NCI)
cancer.gov/about-cancer/treatment/clinical-trials/search

Worldwide

The U.S. National Library of Medicine (NLM)
clinicaltrials.gov

Need help finding a clinical trial?

NCI's Cancer Information Service (CIS)
1.800.4.CANCER (1.800.422.6237)
cancer.gov/contact

Who can enroll?

It depends on the clinical trial's rules, called eligibility criteria. The rules may be about age, cancer type and stage, treatment history, or general health. They ensure that participants are alike in specific ways and that the trial is as safe as possible for the participants.

Informed consent

Clinical trials are managed by a research team. This group of experts will review the study with you in detail, including its purpose and the risks and benefits of joining. All of this information is also provided in an informed consent form. Read the form carefully and ask questions before signing it. Take time to discuss it with people you trust. Keep in mind that you can leave and seek treatment outside of the clinical trial at any time.

Will I get a placebo?

Placebos (inactive versions of real medicines) are almost never used alone in cancer clinical trials. It is common to receive either a placebo with a standard treatment, or a new drug with a standard treatment. You will be informed, verbally and in writing, if a placebo is part of a clinical trial before you enroll.

Are clinical trials free?

There is no fee to enroll in a clinical trial. The study sponsor pays for research-related costs, including the study drug. But you may need to pay for other services, like transportation or childcare, due to extra appointments. During the trial, you will continue to receive standard cancer care. This care is often covered by insurance.

What's next

This chapter explained the many types of treatment available for basal cell skin cancer. The next chapter details treatment that is based on your risk of the cancer's recurrence (returning), called risk status. You will learn what it means if you have low-risk, high-risk, or advanced basal cell skin cancer.

Key points

- Treatments for basal cell skin cancer aim to remove the cancer completely.
- Surgical excision removes the basal cell lesion as well as some normal-looking tissue surrounding it (surgical margin).
- Mohs surgery is commonly used to remove a lesion from the skin.
- Curettage and electrodesiccation is a procedure that removes shallow skin cancers and pre-cancers.
- Radiation therapy uses low-energy photons or electron beam radiation to target cancer cells while minimizing damage to deeper tissues.
- Systemic therapies affect the whole body and can be used for more advanced basal cell skin cancers.

Questions to ask

- How soon do I need to be treated?
- Where will I receive treatment?
- What are the long- and short-term side effects of treatment?
- Should I be aware of any complications?
- What are the expected outcomes of my treatment?

4

Treatment by risk and recurrence

Treatment for basal cell skin cancer is based on the risk of it returning (called recurrence) and, in rare cases, the extent it has spread. This chapter discusses testing and risk status, then presents treatment options based on the specific type of basal cell skin cancer.

The previous chapter described the many types of treatment available for basal cell skin cancer. Which treatment you'll have depends on your risk status. Risk status is an estimate of the likelihood that your cancer will return. In this chapter, you will learn what it means if you have low-risk, high-risk, or advanced basal cell skin cancer.

Testing and diagnosis

Whether you or your doctor found an unusual lesion on your skin, testing is needed to identify and diagnose basal cell skin cancer. As mentioned in *Chapter 2*, this will include a physical exam and medical history to check for specific signs or symptoms as well as a biopsy. But if the lesion is small and shallow enough, your doctor might perform a shave removal. This procedure completely removes the lesion as part of the biopsy.

After the biopsy or shave removal is complete, it is sent to a lab and examined by a pathologist. The information from it will be sent to your doctor in a pathology report. It should detail the risk of the lesion spreading or returning.

Once you are diagnosed with basal cell skin cancer, you will have a complete skin exam to look for other lesions. It's uncommon for basal cell skin cancer to spread. But if the lesion is left untreated, it may grow deeper and wider into surrounding tissues.

Risk status

Basal cell skin cancer is classified by the risk of the cancer coming back after treatment (recurrence). Your risk will be defined based on information from pathology results, where the tumor is located, and how it appears during the skin exam.

Risk is broken up into 3 categories:

- Low risk
- High risk
- Advanced

Low risk

Low-risk basal cell skin cancer means the cancer has a low risk of coming back. Low-risk basal cell skin cancer is defined by the following factors:

- Found on the trunk, arms, or legs
- Small and superficial (found only on top layer of skin)
- Less than 2 centimeters
- Clear, defined edge
- Has not been treated before

High risk

High-risk basal cell skin cancer means there is a higher chance of the cancer coming back after treatment. High-risk basal cell skin cancer is defined by the following factors:

- Found on areas of the face (including eyelids, nose, and lips), head (including ears), neck, arms, hands, trunk, legs, feet, and sometimes the genital area
- Size can be equal to or wider than 2 centimeters
- Poorly defined edge
- Has previously come back after treatment
- Shows an aggressive growth pattern under the microscope

2 centimeters is about the length of a peanut without its shell.

Advanced disease

Advanced basal cell skin cancer means that the lesion has spread either locally (in the surrounding area); regionally (to the lymph nodes, also called nodal); or it has metastasized (to distant areas of the body). If you're diagnosed with advanced disease, you will likely receive imaging before treatment to see how far your cancer has spread.

"I was fortunate I had my basal cell skin cancer successfully removed in its early stages. But I wished I had asked more questions before the Mohs surgery. Even though it's not noticeable as time goes on, I didn't realize how big the scar from surgery can be at the beginning."

High-risk sites for basal cell

Basal cell skin cancer is considered high risk when it is found on the face.

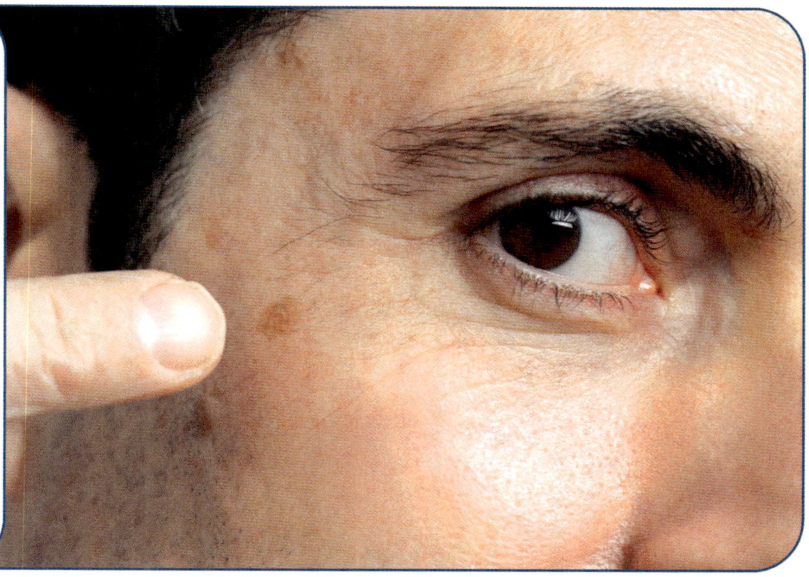

Treatment for low risk

Low-risk basal cell skin cancer is thought to have a low chance of coming back once it's treated. Its location, size, and how well-defined its borders are help determine its risk.

There are many treatment options for low-risk basal cell skin cancer. **See Guide 3**. They include:

- Curettage and electrodesiccation
- Shave removal
- Surgical excision
- Radiation therapy when surgery is not an option
- Topical (nonsurgical) treatments for superficial (shallow) basal cell skin cancer

Guide 3
Possible treatments for low-risk basal cell skin cancer

Curettage and electrodesiccation
Shave removal
Surgical excision
Radiation therapy when surgery is not an option
Topical (nonsurgical) treatments for superficial (shallow) basal cell skin cancer

Curettage and electrodesiccation

Curettage and electrodesiccation is the recommended treatment option for shallow (superficial, affecting the top layer of the skin), low-risk basal cell skin cancer. During the procedure, your doctor will inject a local anesthetic into the affected area to numb it. Then, the lesion will be removed by scraping it with a special tool called a curette that has a sharp looped edge on one side. Next, the doctor will cauterize it and cover it with a bandage, so no stitches are necessary. Still, there's a chance that during the procedure, the lesion may be found to be deeper. If that happens, it might need a surgical excision as a next step.

Shave removal

In this procedure, your doctor will use a sharp blade to remove a shallow lesion, which is at or just below the level of the surrounding skin. A shave removal does not require stitches. But if the lesion is deeper than expected, a standard surgical excision may be needed to remove the remaining cancerous tissue.

Surgical excision

Surgical excision is a primary treatment option for low-risk basal cell skin cancers, especially for those found on the chest, back, hands, and feet. Surgical excision removes the lesion as well as some normal-looking tissue surrounding it (surgical margin). It involves stitches to close the wound. The lesion will be sent to the lab for the pathologist to examine.

If cancer cells are found in the surrounding tissue removed with the tumor (positive margins), more treatment is needed (see *When more treatment is needed*).

Radiation therapy

Radiation therapy can be used when surgery is not an option due to the lesion's location, the person's health status, or if they decline surgery. It typically uses electrons or low-energy radiation to kill or stop cancer cells from growing and minimize damage to deeper tissues. After radiation therapy, you will move to follow-up care (see *Follow-up*).

Topical (nonsurgical) treatments

If your basal cell skin cancer is considered shallow (superficial) and doesn't extend to the dermis, a topical treatment might be a good option. Imiquimod (Aldara) is the preferred topical therapy. Preferred therapies are those that have the most evidence they work better and may be safer than other therapies.

Basal cell skin cancer is highly treatable and curable.

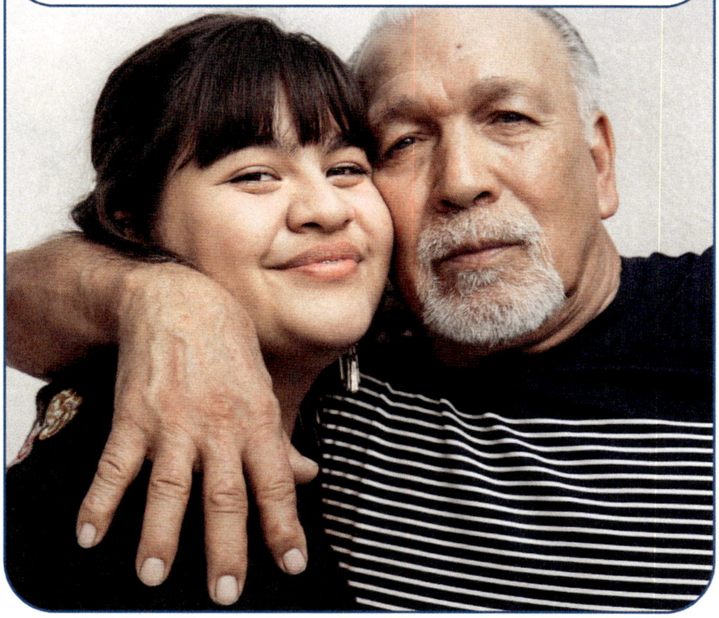

Topical treatment options include:

- Imiquimod (Aldara)
- 5-fluorouracil (Efudex)
- Photodynamic therapy – a topical drug activated by light to kill cancer cells
- Cryotherapy – freezing the lesion with liquid nitrogen through a spray device

After you receive topical treatment, you will move to the follow-up phase of treatment (see *Follow-up*).

When more treatment is needed

If you have surgery to remove low-risk basal cell skin cancer, and no cancer cells are found in the surgical margins (negative margins), then you are ready for follow-up treatment (see *Follow-up*).

But if you have surgery, and there is still remaining cancer (positive margins), you'll need further treatment. Options for the next treatment include:

- Mohs surgery or another form of PDEMA
- Another surgical excision (if possible)
- Radiation therapy (if surgery is not an option and a radiation oncologist helps determine it's appropriate)

After surgery or radiation, you will move to the follow-up phase of treatment (see *Follow-up*).

Treatment for high risk

High-risk basal cell skin cancer means there is a higher chance of the cancer coming back (recurrence) after treatment. Lesions found on the face, head, neck, hands, feet, or shins are at high risk of recurrence, regardless of their size. Lesions on the trunk, other parts of the legs, or arms that are larger than 2 centimeters are also considered high risk. Additionally, lesions with unclear or undefined borders are more likely to recur.

Surgery is often the treatment for high-risk basal cell skin cancer. **See Guide 4**. Two types of surgery are available:

- Mohs surgery or another form of PDEMA (preferred)
- Surgical excision

Mohs surgery

Mohs surgery or other forms of PDEMA are the preferred treatment for high-risk basal cell skin cancer. Preferred treatments are those that have the most evidence they work better and may be safer than other treatments.

Guide 4 Treatment options for high-risk basal cell skin cancer
Mohs surgery or other forms of PDEMA
Surgical excision with wider margins
Discussion with care team, including radiation oncologist, about radiation therapy

Mohs surgery removes tumors from the skin, layer by layer. If there are additional areas of concern around the edges or base of the tissue sample, you will have another round of tissue removal. You will continue this process until all the affected tissue has been removed and surgical margins are clear (negative for cancer). At that point, you will move to follow-up care (see *Follow-up*).

Even if Mohs surgery is successful and the margins are clear, radiation therapy might be added if cancer cells are found in or around nerves, or if there are concerning microscopic findings. Otherwise, you will move to follow-up care (see *Follow-up*).

Surgical excision

A surgical excision with wider surgical margins is recommended for high-risk basal cell skin cancer. A wider surgical margin refers to the area of normal tissue removed around the lesion. After the procedure, it will be tested to find out if the surgery removed all of the cancer cells. If successful, you will move to follow-up care. If testing finds cancer in the margin (a positive margin), more treatment is needed.

Additional treatment

If surgery doesn't remove all the cancer, you and your care team will discuss what treatment comes next. Treatment at this point may include another surgery or radiation therapy. If another surgery can be performed, this is generally tried first. Otherwise, radiation therapy is used. If either treatment is successful in eliminating the cancer, you will move to follow-up care.

If you've had surgery and/or radiation therapy, and cancer is still present, then your cancer will be classified as advanced basal cell skin cancer (see *Treatment for advanced disease*).

When surgery is not an option

But if surgery is not an option for you, your doctor will likely consult with different members of your care team to talk with you about next steps. This team should include a radiation oncologist to discuss using radiation therapy to treat your lesion.

Treatment for advanced disease

Basal cell skin cancer rarely spreads (metastasizes). But if the lesion goes untreated, it may spread. When it does occur, you will have imaging first to help determine how deep and far your skin cancer has spread. Next, your doctor and your care team will meet with you about your treatment. If radiation therapy is considered, a radiation oncologist should work with you and your care team to decide if it's right for you. **See Guide 5**.

Guide 5 **Treatment options for advanced basal cell skin cancer**
Surgery (Mohs, PDEMA, or standard excision)
Radiation therapy
Systemic therapy
Clinical trial
Supportive care

What makes someone not eligible for surgery?

Some people with basal cell skin cancer are not candidates for surgery. What this means is that surgery won't be recommended as a treatment. Some of the reasons surgery is not recommended could include one or more of the following:

- **Difficult location** – If the lesion is in a spot that's tricky or risky for surgery, like near the eyes, ears, or nose
- **Large or deep lesions** – If the lesion is very large or has grown deep into the skin, making it hard to remove completely
- **Health concerns** – If a person has other health issues or if they're older, making surgery risky
- **Recurrence** – If the cancer has come back or hasn't responded well to surgery in the past
- **Nerve invasion** – If the cancer has spread along the nerves, making it harder to remove with surgery

Treatment includes several options depending on which of the 3 types of advanced basal cell skin cancer you have:

- Locally advanced or unresectable disease, which means it has spread deep into the skin or surrounding area making surgery (also called resection) more difficult
- Nodal (or regional) disease, which means it has spread to the lymph nodes
- Metastatic disease, which means it has spread far from the original lesion to another area of the body

Locally advanced or unresectable disease

Locally advanced means the cancer has spread deeper into the skin or nearby tissues. It can be large, aggressive, or a lesion that has come back. Unresectable disease means the lesion can't be fully removed by surgery.

Because the cancer is more advanced, you may receive neoadjuvant systemic therapy first. This may be with the drug vismodegib, which is a targeted therapy. In some cases, you might receive cemiplimab-rwlc, which is an immunotherapy.

For the treatment of locally advanced disease, you have the following options:

- Another surgery – Mohs or another kind of PDEMA is preferable but if they are not available, standard excision surgery is an option.
- Radiation therapy

What is PDEMA?

Peripheral and deep en face margin assessment (PDEMA) is a technique that lets your doctor see the entire edge of removed tissue clearly.

This is also called a complete margin assessment. Mohs surgery is one type of PDEMA.

- If neither surgery nor radiation therapy are an option, then systemic therapy would be recommended. This includes targeted therapies or in some cases, immunotherapy.

Treatment using systemic therapies

Systemic therapies are cancer treatments that affect the whole body. Targeted therapies and immunotherapies can be used for advanced basal cell skin cancer when other treatments are not an option.

- **Vismodegib** (Erivedge) – Vismodegib is a targeted therapy and may be used for locally advanced, nodal (regional), or metastatic basal cell skin cancer. It can be used as a primary treatment for those who cannot have surgery or radiation, or if there are cancer cells found after surgery and surgery is no longer possible.
- **Sonidegib** (Odomzo) – Sonidegib is a targeted therapy. It may be used to treat people with locally advanced or nodal (regional) basal cell skin cancer that has recurred following surgery or

radiation therapy, or for those who are not candidates for surgery or radiation therapy.

- **Cemiplimab-rwlc** (Libtayo) – Cemiplimab-rwlc is an immunotherapy agent that is sometimes used to treat locally advanced, nodal (regional), or metastatic basal cell skin cancer. It is used if the cancer worsens after using vismodegib or sonidegib, or if you are unable to take those therapies.

Nodal (or regional) disease

Nodal disease means cancer has spread regionally to the lymph nodes. Lymph nodes are small bean-shaped structures that help fight infection and disease. When skin cancer spreads from the original tumor to the lymph nodes, this can signal that the cancer is more advanced and may have spread to other parts of the body through the lymphatic system. Still, this type of spread is very rare.

When cancer is in the lymph nodes, your treatment options include:

- Surgery with or without radiation therapy after surgery (called adjuvant radiation).
- If surgery is not an option, then radiation therapy or systemic therapy with targeted therapy (vismodegib or sonidegib), or, in some cases, immunotherapy (cemiplimab-rwlc)
- Treatment in a clinical trial

Metastatic disease

Metastatic disease means the cancer has spread to distant parts of the body. This type of spread is extremely rare. If your basal cell skin cancer is considered metastatic, your doctor and care team will discuss with you your best course of action. Depending on the cancer's spread, your treatment may include any of the following:

- Systemic therapy with vismodegib or, in some cases, cemiplimab-rwlc
- Radiation therapy or surgery for limited metastatic disease
- Palliative care, which is also known as supportive care (see *Supportive care*)

Advanced basal cell skin cancer is rare. Still, there are many treatment options.

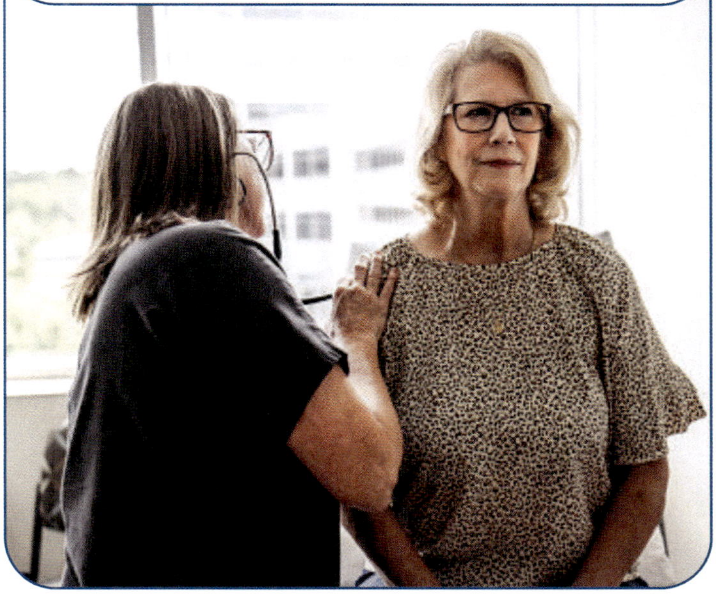

Follow-up

During the follow-up phase of your treatment, your care team will closely monitor you for any new skin lesions and talk to you about prevention. Having basal cell skin cancer increases your risk for other types of skin cancer, like squamous cell carcinoma and melanoma, so these exams are very important.

You will have a complete skin exam every 6 to 12 months for the first 5 years, and then at least once a year for life. Imaging tests to get more information about any concerning lesions might be needed. If there's suspicion that your basal cell skin cancer has come back, closely follow your care team's advice on what to do next.

Finding basal cell skin cancer early when it is easier to treat is ideal. And you can do this on your own. Between follow-up visits, check your skin regularly. If you notice anything unusual, see your doctor as soon as possible. For all skin cancers, the sooner you find and treat them, the better it is for you and your health.

"I spent my childhood in the sun and back then, there was very little understanding of the damage it can cause. Now, as an adult who was treated for basal cell skin cancer, I make sure I wear sunscreen every day, all year long."

Prevention

While there is no proven way to prevent skin cancer, you may be able to lower your risk of future skin cancers. Speak with your doctor about your risk.

Taking the following steps may help reduce your risk:

Reduce UV light exposure

This means reducing exposure to the sun and avoiding the use of indoor tanning beds.

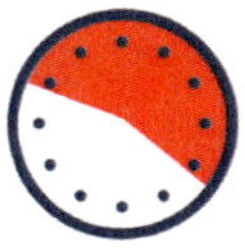

Prevent sun damage

Limit sun exposure between peak hours of 10:00 AM and 4:00 PM.

Wear protective clothing

This includes a wide-brimmed hat, clothes made with UV-protective fabric, and sunglasses.

Use sunscreen

Choose a broad-spectrum sunscreen with a sun protection factor (SPF) of at least 30 and reapply every 2 hours. Sunscreen should also be applied 15 minutes before going outside.

Examine your skin regularly

This includes self-examinations with the assistance of a partner and skin exams by a health care provider.

Treatment for recurrence

Once you are in follow-up care and you're monitored closely, if you or your doctor sees a return of your lesion, then that is called recurrence. **See Guide 6**. There are two types of recurrence: Local or advanced disease.

Local disease

Local disease means that the cancer has returned at or near the same spot. Local disease is usually treated with surgery (Mohs or surgical excision with wider margins). But if surgery is not an option for you, your doctor will likely consult other team members that should include a radiation oncologist to determine if you should have radiation therapy.

Advanced disease

If cancer has spread to nearby lymph nodes or to distant parts of the body (metastasized), it's considered an advanced recurrence. In this case, your doctor will discuss the best next steps for your treatment with your care team.

Treatment options for advanced recurrence include:

- Surgery for locally advanced, nodal, or limited metastatic disease
- Radiation therapy (if surgery was not possible or given after surgery)
- Systemic therapy (either before surgery, if surgery and radiation therapy were not successful, or if surgery is not possible)
- Clinical trial for nodal disease
- Supportive care for metastatic disease

Supportive care

Supportive care helps improve your quality of life during and after cancer treatment.

The goal is to prevent or manage side effects and symptoms, like pain and cancer-related fatigue. It also addresses the mental, social, and spiritual concerns faced by those with cancer.

Supportive care is available to everyone with cancer and their families, not just those at the end of life. Palliative care is another name for supportive care.

Supportive care can also help with:

- Making treatment decisions
- Coordinating your care
- Paying for care
- Planning for advanced care and end of life

Guide 6 Treatment options for basal cell skin cancer recurrence
Surgery (Mohs, PDEMA, or standard excision)
Radiation therapy
Systemic therapy
Clinical trial
Supportive care

Key points

- Surgery is the most common treatment for all basal cell skin cancer.
- High-risk basal cell skin cancer means there is a higher chance of the cancer coming back after treatment.
- Advanced basal cell skin cancer, which means it has spread locally or distantly, is not common.
- After primary treatment is finished, you will be monitored for cancer that may return called recurrence.
- If cancer returns at or near the same place, it is called a local disease recurrence.
- If cancer spreads to lymph nodes or distant parts of the body, it is called advanced disease recurrence.
- Expect to receive a complete skin exam every 6 to 12 months for the first 5 years, and then annually for life.

Questions to ask

- Are there any complications from treatment?
- Will I need reconstructive surgery?
- What is the chance for recurrence?
- Am I eligible for a clinical trial?
- How often will I need follow-up visits after I finish treatment?

"I had my first Mohs surgery in my early 30s and have had a few more since then for both basal and squamous cell skin cancers. I'm a runner and worked as a lifeguard in my youth — not great activities for a fair skinned, blue-eyed person. Even though I covered my nose in white zinc oxide when working at the pool, the rest of my body fried and now in my 60s, I'm paying the price. Still, I'm so thankful for my dermatologist and Mohs surgery."

5
Other resources

Want to learn more? Here's how you can get additional help.

What else to know

This book can help you improve your basal cell skin cancer care. It plainly explains expert recommendations and suggests questions to ask your care team. But it's not the only resource that you have.

You're welcome to receive as much information and help as you need. Many people are interested in learning more about:

- The details of their health and treatment
- Being a part of a care team
- Getting financial help
- Finding a care provider who is an expert in their field
- Coping with health problems

What else to do

Your health care center can help you with next steps. They often have on-site resources to help meet your needs and find answers to your questions. Health care centers can also inform you of resources in your community.

In addition to help from your providers, the resources listed in the next section provide support for many people like yourself. Look through the list and visit the provided websites to learn more about these organizations.

Where to get help

Aim at Skin Cancer
AIMatSkinCancer.org

Cancer*Care*
Cancercare.org

Cancer Hope Network
Cancerhopenetwork.org

Imerman Angels
Imermanangels.org

National Coalition for Cancer Survivorship
canceradvocacy.org

Save Your Skin Foundation
saveyourskin.ca

Triage Cancer
triagecancer.org

Questions to ask

- Can I get a second opinion?
- What will happen if I do nothing?
- Can you help me learn more about clinical trials?

Words to know

basal cell carcinoma (BCC)
Also known as basal cell skin cancer, it is a type of skin cancer that most often develops on areas of skin exposed to the sun, such as the face.

best supportive care
Treatment given to prevent, control, or relieve side effects and improve comfort and quality of life.

biopsy
Removal of small amounts of tissue from your body to test for disease.

broad-spectrum sunscreen
A substance that protects the skin from the sun by blocking 2 types of harmful ultraviolet (UV) rays — UVA and UVB.

chemotherapy
Drugs that kill fast-growing cells, including normal cells and cancer cells.

clinical trial
Research on a test or treatment to assess its safety or how well it works.

computed tomography (CT) scan
A test that takes x-rays from different angles to create an image of the inside of the body.

dermatologist
A doctor who's an expert in skin diseases.

dermis
The second layer of skin that is beneath the top layer (epidermis).

epidermis
The outer layer of skin.

excision
Removal by surgery.

follow-up
The time after treatment where you see your doctor on a routine basis for monitoring of your condition.

intravenous (IV)
A method of giving drugs by a needle or tube inserted into a vein.

local anesthetic
A temporary loss of feeling in one small area of the body caused by special drugs called anesthetics.

locally advanced
When the basal cell skin cancer has spread deeper into the skin or nearby tissues.

magnetic resonance imaging (MRI)
A test that uses radio waves and powerful magnets to view the inside of the body.

metastasize
When cancer cells spread to a part of the body away from the first (primary) tumor.

nodal disease
Cancer cells that have spread from the primary tumor, regionally, to the lymph nodes.

palliative care
Specialized medical care aimed at increasing quality of life and reducing pain and discomfort for people with serious, complex illness.

PDEMA
A peripheral and deep en face margin assessment (PDEMA) refers to a technique that allows your doctor to view a high-quality

image of the entire marginal surface of removed tissues.

resectable
A tumor able to be removed (resected) by surgery.

shave removal
A procedure where the doctor uses a sharp blade to remove a shallow lesion, which is at or below the level of the surrounding skin.

sun protection factor (SPF)
A rating of protection against ultraviolet rays.

surgical margin
The normal, healthy-looking tissue that was removed around a tumor during surgery.

systemic therapy
Treatment using substances that travel through the bloodstream, reaching and affecting cells all over the body.

unresectable
Not capable of being surgically removed.

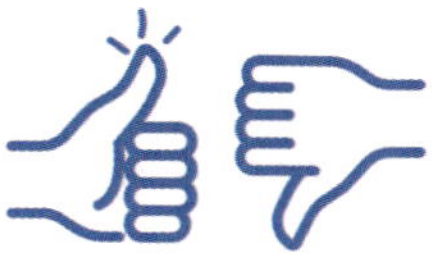

Let us know what you think!

Please take a moment to complete an online survey about the NCCN Guidelines for Patients.

NCCN.org/patients/response

NCCN Contributors

This patient guide is based on the NCCN Clinical Practice Guidelines in Oncology (NCCN Guidelines®) for Basal Cell Skin Cancer, Version 1.2025. It was adapted, reviewed, and published with help from the following people:

Dorothy A. Shead, MS
Senior Director
Patient Information Operations

Christine McLaughlin
Medical Writer

Susan Kidney
Senior Graphic Design Specialist

The NCCN Clinical Practice Guidelines in Oncology (NCCN Guidelines®) for Basal Cell Skin Cancer, Version 1.2025 were developed by the following NCCN Panel Members:

Jeremy Bordeaux, MD, MPH/Chair
Case Comprehensive Cancer Center/ University Hospitals Seidman Cancer Center and Cleveland Clinic Taussig Cancer Institute

Rachel Blitzblau, MD, PhD/ Vice Chair
Duke Cancer Institute

Sumaira Z. Aasi, MD
Stanford Cancer Institute

Murad Alam, MD, MBA, MSCI
Robert H. Lurie Comprehensive Cancer Center of Northwestern University

*Arya Amini, MD
City of Hope National Medical Center

Kristin Bibee, MD, PhD
Johns Hopkins Kimmel Cancer Center

Diana Bolotin, MD, PhD
The UChicago Medicine Comprehensive Cancer Center

Pei-Ling Chen, MD, PhD
Moffitt Cancer Center

Carlo M. Contreras, MD
The Ohio State University Comprehensive Cancer Center - James Cancer Hospital and Solove Research Institute

Dominick DiMaio, MD
Fred & Pamela Buffett Cancer Center

Jessica M. Donigan, MD
Huntsman Cancer Institute at the University of Utah

*Daniel Eisen, MD
UC Davis Comprehensive Cancer Center

Jeffrey M. Farma, MD
Fox Chase Cancer Center

Karthik Ghosh, MD
Mayo Clinic Comprehensive Cancer Center

Kelly Harms, MD, PhD
University of Michigan Rogel Cancer Center

Nicole LeBoeuf, MD, MPH
Dana-Farber/Brigham and Women's Cancer Center | Mass General Cancer Center

John Nicholas Lukens, MD
Abramson Cancer Center at the University of Pennsylvania

*Susan Manber
Publicis Health

Lawrence Mark, MD, PhD
Indiana University Melvin and Bren Simon Comprehensive Cancer Center

Stacy McMurray, MD
Vanderbilt-Ingram Cancer Center

Theresa Medina, MD
University of Colorado Cancer Center

Kishwer S. Nehal, MD
Memorial Sloan Kettering Cancer Center

Paul Nghiem, MD, PhD
Fred Hutchinson Cancer Center

Kelly Olino, MD
Yale Cancer Center/Smilow Cancer Hospital

Gyorgy Paragh, MD, PhD
Roswell Park Comprehensive Cancer Center

Soo Park, MD
UC San Diego Moores Cancer Center

Tejesh Patel, MD
The University of Tennessee Health Science Center

Jason Rich, MD
Siteman Cancer Center at Barnes-Jewish Hospital and Washington University School of Medicine

Ashok R. Shaha, MD
Memorial Sloan Kettering Cancer Center

Bhavina Sharma, MD, MPH
Fred & Pamela Buffett Cancer Center

Yemi Sokumbi, MD
Mayo Clinic Comprehensive Cancer Center

Divya Srivastava, MD
UT Southwestern Simmons Comprehensive Cancer Center

Joel Sunshine, MD, PhD
Johns Hopkins Kimmel Cancer Center

Valencia Thomas, MD
The University of Texas MD Anderson Cancer Center

Courtney Tomblinson, MD
Vanderbilt-Ingram Cancer Center

Puja Venkat, MD
UCLA Jonsson Comprehensive Cancer Center

Yaohui Gloria Xu, MD, PhD
University of Wisconsin Carbone Cancer Center

Siegrid Yu, MD
UCSF Helen Diller Family Comprehensive Cancer Center

*Mehran Yusuf, MD
O'Neal Comprehensive Cancer Center at UAB

NCCN

Sara Espinosa, PhD
Oncology Scientist, Medical Writer

Beth McCullough, RN, BS
Guidelines Coordinator

* Reviewed this patient guide.
For disclosures, visit NCCN.org/disclosures.

NCCN Cancer Centers

Abramson Cancer Center
at the University of Pennsylvania
Philadelphia, Pennsylvania
800.789.7366 • pennmedicine.org/cancer

Case Comprehensive Cancer Center/
University Hospitals Seidman Cancer Center and
Cleveland Clinic Taussig Cancer Institute
Cleveland, Ohio
UH Seidman Cancer Center
800.641.2422 • uhhospitals.org/services/cancer-services
CC Taussig Cancer Institute
866.223.8100 • my.clevelandclinic.org/departments/cancer
Case CCC
216.844.8797 • case.edu/cancer

City of Hope National Medical Center
Duarte, California
800.826.4673 • cityofhope.org

Dana-Farber/Brigham and Women's Cancer Center |
Mass General Cancer Center
Boston, Massachusetts
877.442.3324 • youhaveus.org
617.726.5130 • massgeneral.org/cancer-center

Duke Cancer Institute
Durham, North Carolina
888.275.3853 • dukecancerinstitute.org

Fox Chase Cancer Center
Philadelphia, Pennsylvania
888.369.2427 • foxchase.org

Fred & Pamela Buffett Cancer Center
Omaha, Nebraska
402.559.5600 • unmc.edu/cancercenter

Fred Hutchinson Cancer Center
Seattle, Washington
206.667.5000 • fredhutch.org

Huntsman Cancer Institute at the University of Utah
Salt Lake City, Utah
800.824.2073 • healthcare.utah.edu/huntsmancancerinstitute

Indiana University Melvin and Bren Simon
Comprehensive Cancer Center
Indianapolis, Indiana
888.600.4822 • www.cancer.iu.edu

Johns Hopkins Kimmel Cancer Center
Baltimore, Maryland
410.955.8964
www.hopkinskimmelcancercenter.org

Mayo Clinic Comprehensive Cancer Center
Phoenix/Scottsdale, Arizona
Jacksonville, Florida
Rochester, Minnesota
480.301.8000 • Arizona
904.953.0853 • Florida
507.538.3270 • Minnesota
mayoclinic.org/cancercenter

Memorial Sloan Kettering Cancer Center
New York, New York
800.525.2225 • mskcc.org

Moffitt Cancer Center
Tampa, Florida
888.663.3488 • moffitt.org

O'Neal Comprehensive Cancer Center at UAB
Birmingham, Alabama
800.822.0933 • uab.edu/onealcancercenter

Robert H. Lurie Comprehensive Cancer Center
of Northwestern University
Chicago, Illinois
866.587.4322 • cancer.northwestern.edu

Roswell Park Comprehensive Cancer Center
Buffalo, New York
877.275.7724 • roswellpark.org

Siteman Cancer Center at Barnes-Jewish Hospital
and Washington University School of Medicine
St. Louis, Missouri
800.600.3606 • siteman.wustl.edu

St. Jude Children's Research Hospital/
The University of Tennessee Health Science Center
Memphis, Tennessee
866.278.5833 • stjude.org
901.448.5500 • uthsc.edu

Stanford Cancer Institute
Stanford, California
877.668.7535 • cancer.stanford.edu

The Ohio State University Comprehensive Cancer Center -
James Cancer Hospital and Solove Research Institute
Columbus, Ohio
800.293.5066 • cancer.osu.edu

The UChicago Medicine Comprehensive Cancer Center
Chicago, Illinois
773.702.1000 • uchicagomedicine.org/cancer

The University of Texas MD Anderson Cancer Center
Houston, Texas
844.269.5922 • mdanderson.org

UC Davis Comprehensive Cancer Center
Sacramento, California
916.734.5959 • 800.770.9261
health.ucdavis.edu/cancer

UC San Diego Moores Cancer Center
La Jolla, California
858.822.6100 • cancer.ucsd.edu

UCLA Jonsson Comprehensive Cancer Center
Los Angeles, California
310.825.5268 • uclahealth.org/cancer

UCSF Helen Diller Family
Comprehensive Cancer Center
San Francisco, California
800.689.8273 • cancer.ucsf.edu

University of Colorado Cancer Center
Aurora, Colorado
720.848.0300 • coloradocancercenter.org

University of Michigan Rogel Cancer Center
Ann Arbor, Michigan
800.865.1125 • rogelcancercenter.org

University of Wisconsin Carbone Cancer Center
Madison, Wisconsin
608.265.1700 • uwhealth.org/cancer

UT Southwestern Simmons
Comprehensive Cancer Center
Dallas, Texas
214.648.3111 • utsouthwestern.edu/simmons

Vanderbilt-Ingram Cancer Center
Nashville, Tennessee
877.936.8422 • vicc.org

Yale Cancer Center/Smilow Cancer Hospital
New Haven, Connecticut
855.4.SMILOW • yalecancercenter.org

share with us.

Take our survey and help make the NCCN Guidelines for Patients better for everyone!

NCCN.org/patients/comments

Notes

Index

Made in the USA
Coppell, TX
05 January 2026

68260448R00029